# The Little Book of Yoga Meditation

## Scott Shaw

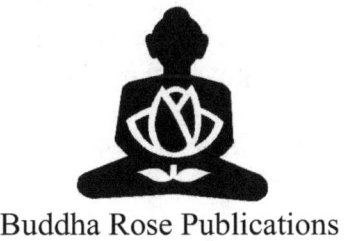

Buddha Rose Publications

The Little Book of Yoga Meditation
www.scottshaw.com
Copyright © 2013
ALL RIGHTS RESERVED

First Edition

ISBN 10: 1-877792-67-5
ISBN 13: 9781877792670

Library of Congress Control Number: 2013935002

This book contains material protected under International and Federal Copyright Laws and Treaties. Any unauthorized reprint or use of this material is prohibited. No part of this book may be reproduced or transmitted in any form or by any means, electronic or mechanical, including photocopying, recording, or by any information storage and retrieval system without express written permission from the author or publisher.

Disclaimer: The author and the publishers of this book are in no way responsible, in any manner whatsoever, for any injury that may result from practicing the techniques presented in this text. Since the practices discussed in this book may be too strenuous for some readers, it is highly suggested that you consult your physician before you undertake any physical activities.

10 9 8 7 6 5 4 3 2 1
Printed in the United States of America

# The Little Book of
# *Yoga Meditation*

# Table of Contents

|    | | |
|----|--|--|
|    | Introduction | 7 |
| 1  | Raja Yoga | 9 |
| 2  | Astanga Yoga | 13 |
| 3  | Yama | 15 |
| 4  | Niyama | 19 |
| 5  | Asana: The Seat of Meditation | 25 |
| 6  | Pranayama: Breath Control | 27 |
| 7  | Pratyahara | 33 |
| 8  | Dharana | 37 |
| 9  | Dhyana | 45 |
| 10 | Mudra | 47 |
| 11 | Meditative Focus | 51 |
| 12 | Mantra | 53 |
| 13 | Brahmamurti | 61 |
| 14 | Samadhi | 63 |
|    | Conclusion | 65 |
|    | About the Author | 67 |
|    | Scott Shaw: Books-in-Print | 69 |

# Introduction

The fast pace of the modern world has left people separated from a sense of mental and physical well-being. These factors have caused many to turn to all type of antidotes. There is caffeinated drinks to amplify one's metabolism. There are prescription and nonprescription drugs designed to calm a person down. But, no matter what the source of these cure-alls, they all have one thing in common – they are not natural. There is, however, an ancient method designed to bring the body and the mind of the individual into a natural state of calm and harmony. That method is meditation.

The techniques of meditation have been acutely defined in the ancient practice of yoga. The word, *"Yoga"* is commonly attributed solely to physical postures associated with this age-old science. But, yoga is much more than this. Yoga is a Sanskrit word that means, *"Joining"* or *"Union."* The techniques of yoga meditation are, therefore, ideally designed to bring about a conscious unity of body, mind, and spirit to the practitioner.

But, what exactly is yoga meditation? When you mention the word meditation to the layperson, the vision of a monk with their mind locked deeply into communion with the abstract realms of *Cosmic Consciousness* is oftentimes the thought that is brought to mind. Though this is how meditation has been depicted, this is not the ultimate definition of meditation.

Meditation is available to everyone – not simply a monk living in a monastery. Yoga meditation is a simple and refined group of practices designed to focus the mind of the practitioner to the degree that they can consciously tune-out the distractions of the modern world and bring themselves into a calmer and more conscious state of harmony with their body, their mind, and the external world. To achieve this, the practitioner of yoga meditation embraces a refined group of mental practices known in Sanskrit as, *"Sadhana." Sadhana* or *"Spiritual Exercises,"* are designed to purify the body and the mind of the practitioner and lead them towards a state of true mental calm and meditation.

The techniques designed for the practice of yoga meditation were ideally defined by the branch of yoga known as *Raja Yoga*. R*aja Yoga* is the category of yoga where the practitioner learns to refine their mental consciousness, thereby easily embrace the practice of meditation.

Throughout the pages of this book, the techniques and philosophic ideologies of *Raja Yoga* will be detailed in order to provide you with a firm foundation in order for you to enter into the realms of yoga meditation. From this, you may hopefully enter into a new, calmer, a more refined life, where the obstacles of the modern world no longer control you and cause you to lose your true inner peace.

# Chapter 1
# Raja Yoga

*Raja Yoga* is translated as, *"The King's Yoga."* This terminology is not used to imply that only those of aristocratic decent can practice this form of yoga. Instead, it delineates that Raja Yoga is the royal or higher-path to body and mind unification.

*Raja Yoga* is a mental pathway. The techniques of *Raja Yoga* teach the aspirant to silence the mind in order to come into union with the self and the divine aspects of this universe.

## Defining Human Consciousness

In *Raja Yoga* it is detailed that there are five states of human consciousness. Each of these states defines how an individual behaves while they are dwelling at a certain level of human awareness.

These Five Stages of Raja Yoga are:
1. Kshipta
2. Mudha
3. Vikshipta
4. Ekagra
5. Niruddha

## The Five States of Human Consciousness

To come to better understand how the human mind operates, we can view these five *Raja Yoga* delineations in order to come to possess a better framework of mental understanding in order to more easily enter into the realms of meditation.

1. **Kshipta** defines the state of mental consciousness that the average person possesses. At this level the human mind is running unhindered from one thought onto the next. Here, the emotions are dominated by desires and influenced by sensory perception. The individual has difficultly focusing upon anything but momentary carvings.

2. **Mudha** is the first level that the practitioner of meditation encounters when they have become exposed to the meditative disciplines. At this level the practitioner understands that there is something more to human existence than simply momentary gratification. At this stage the practitioner is attempting to focus his or her mind to the degree where they may delve into deeper knowledge.

Many beginning practitioners of meditation are never able to rise above this level of consciousness due to the fact that they are so controlled by the distraction of the material work. From this, many beginning practitioner of meditation fall away from the practice.

3. **Vikshipta** is the level when the meditation practitioner formally begins to tame their mind. It is at this point, in the ongoing evolution of consciousness that he or she comes to fully understand that they must come into control of their mind, through the techniques of meditation, in order to ascend to the higher levels of human consciousness.

At the stage of *Vikshipta* the practitioner's concentration is quickly lost from the realms of meditation, however, as human desires are still the dominant force in his or her life. Thus, the mind is quickly distracted.

4. *Ekagra* is the state of being that come to exist in the mind of the practitioner through prolonged periods of concentration and meditation. At this level the practitioner reaches a state where he or she becomes one-pointed and focused upon their meditation. At this stage they understand that it is essential to calm and master the mind in order to transcend to the high realms of human consciousness.

5. *Niruddha* is the level where the practitioner of meditation completely silences the mind. At this stage they enter into a state of complete harmony with self and the external universe.

# Chapter 2
## Astanga Yoga

During the second century C.E. a revered East India Sage named Patanjali refocused and redefine the techniques of *Raja Yoga* and meditation. Though very little biographical knowledge exists about this historic figure, his writings helped to refined *Raja Yoga,* making it a much more refined discipline.

During his lifetime, Patanjali defined a process whereby the practitioner of meditation can follow a step-by-step pathway. The teachings of Patanjali are known as *Astanga Yoga. Astanga* is the, *"Eightfold Path of Yoga."*

### The Eightfold Path

Patanjali's *Eightfold Path of Astanga Yoga* precisely defines the steps a practitioner of meditation must pass through in order to obtain complete meditative self-awareness.

**The Eight Stages of Astanga Yoga are:**
1. Yama
2. Niyama
3. Asana
4. Pranayama
5. Pratyahara
6. Dharana
7. Dhyana
8. Samadhi

# Chapter 3
## Yama

The first stage of Patanjali's *Eightfold Path of Astanga Yoga* is Yama. Yama is the formal vows a meditator takes when he or she consciously enters upon the path of meditation. This is the first mindful step that is taken when they decide to leave behind the constraints of *Maya, "This illusionary world,"* purify their mind, and move towards a more refined consciousness. Therefore, *Yama* is the necessary first rung of the eightfold ladder of *Astanga Yoga*.

### The Five Formal Vows

There are five formal vows of *Yama*. These moral observances are known in Sanskrit as, *"Maha Vrata"* or *"The Great Vows."*

### The Five Vows of Yama are:
1. Ahimsa
2. Satya
3. Asteya
4. Brahamcharya
5. Aparigraha

1. ***Ahimsa*** means *"Non-violence."* This understanding is elemental to the aspirant's movements towards true meditative self-awareness. The vows of Ahimsa teach the meditative practitioner to love all things and refrain from confrontation.

The individual on the path of meditation consciousness must not allow him or herself to be drawn into meaningless battles – be they physical, mental, or verbal. This is based upon the understanding that all confrontation simply lead to further confrontation and, thus, confrontations disrupt one meditative consciousness.

**2. Satya** means *"Truth."* This vow details that not only must the meditative practitioner embrace truth in the spoken word but it must be embrace on a metaphysical level, as well.

Many people falsely believe that simply because they believe something to be true, it is true. This type of truth is based upon personal perception. Personal perception is dominated by society, culture, and desire. Therefore this type of belief is not truth. Truth is what remains when all of the temporary illusionary stimuli of this material world are removed from individual perception and the understanding of pure consciousness is embraced. This advance level of consciousness may be embraced in the realms of meditation when the thinking mind is consciously turned off and the pure meditative mind is encountered.

**3. Asteya** means *"Non-stealing."* Much more than simply not being a thief, *Asteya* teaches the meditative practitioner that all actions possess consequences. If you ask a person for a favor, *karma* is created. If you go to somebody expecting him or her to give you something, *karma* is created. If you take something from somebody, *karma* is created.

*Karma* is a very subtle element of human existence. It is most simply defined in the statement, *"As you sew, so shall you reap."* To this end, the understanding of *Asteya* teaches the meditative practitioner to never expect or take anything from another person, unless it is based in absolute spiritual necessity. For if you do, *karma* will be created. If this *karma* is based in a negative action, such as taking something from another individual in a less than spiritual manner, then negative *karma* is created. And, negative *karma* haunts the individual and keeps the person from embracing the pure-mind of meditation.

4. **Brahamcharya**, translated from the Sanskrit means, *"Brahmaic"* or *"God-like conduct."* This term most commonly refers to abstinence from sex – as this practice has traditionally shown that an individual is not lost in the gratification of his or her senses.

*Brahamcharya* is much more than celibacy, however. *Brahamcharya* is the state where the meditative practitioner consciously leaves behind the desires of material existence. This process does not happen instantaneously. Instead, what occurs through the continued clarifying of the mind, via meditation, is that a gradual falling away of the various desires which once dominated your mind takes place – leaving you experiencing fulfillment in a much more substantial fashion than the temporal satisfaction of obtaining material objects and physical conquests.

It is essential to note that *Brahamcharya* does not mean that you are expected to instantaneously be free of desire. Simply by working on clarifying your mind, through the practices of meditation, you will find that you pass through each step of spiritual evolution at your own rate. Each of your desires will fall away when it is their time to leave you.

**5.** *Aparigraha* is the *"Renunciation of greed."* Greed is one of the most damning factors of human existence. Greed for power, money, possessions, and sex dominate many people's entire lives. The uncontrolled desire for spiritual enlightenment is also a form of greed. And, though the individual on the path to enlightenment may believe that he or she is walking the path of God realization, they are, in fact, doing just the opposite. For this reason, Patanjali details that the individual who wished to truly enter into the path of meditation must consciously renounce desire and greed at all levels.

Again, desires are not expected to fall away immediately. And, one should not become mad at themselves when the find they are still desiring certain objects. The path of yoga meditation provided the practitioner with a pathway to ever-evolving consciousness. For this reason, one simply has to practice the techniques of meditation and desire will naturally fall away.

# Chapter 4
## Niyama

*Niyama* is the second stage of Patanjali's Eightfold Path. *Niyama* means *"Restraint."*

As with *Yama*, *Niyama* possesses five prescribed practices that the practitioner of yoga meditation can embrace to continue their personal evolution towards a meditative mindset.

**The Five Stages of Niyama are:**
1. Shauca
2. Samtosha
3. Tapas
4. Svadhyaya
5. Ishvara Pranidhana

1. ***Shauca*** means *"Purity."* To the modern practitioner of meditation, the practice of *Shauca* dictates that you avoid negative people, negative environments, negative food and drink, and consciously attempt to embrace righteous behavior in all of your actions.

Purity is not an external image. It is not the clothing that you wear or the external impression that you project. It is, however, what you say, what you do, and how you behave when interacting with all other entities of this world.

How you behave is your choice. How you react to the way others behave towards you is also your choice. You can choose to be a kind and positive person no matter how negative any person or situation may seem to be. With this, you radiate positive, pure energy to all that you encounter. This is the ideal representation of *Shauca*.

**2. Samtosha** is *"Contentment."* Contentment means that you do not desire anything more than what you already possess, be it physical, material, emotional, or spiritual. With this mindset you instantly embrace the higher essence of the meditative mind. Lacking desire, you are free. Thus, meditation occurs naturally.

Most people unconsciously separate themselves from *Samtosha*. They believe they must look a certain way or behave in a specific fashion in order to suit the people they are attempting to gain love, respect, or acceptance from. This type of false behavior is not solely lost to the material world; it is very common in spiritual communities, as well.

This type of conduct, though very common, is one of the root causes of unhappiness – no matter how hard you try you can not make anyone else happy as long as you are not being true to yourself.

Embracing *Samtosha* witness an individual consciously stopping their attempts to please others.

When you stop judging yourself by comparison with others, you allow your body to be your body, your mind to be your mind, and you to be you. With this comes a normal state of contentment. With this, the practice of meditation is easily entered into.

**3. Tapas**, literally translated from Sanskrit, means *"Heat or Glow."* *Tapas,* also called, *"Tapasia,"* when referring to spiritual practices details, *"Austerities"* or "Asceticism."

It is understood that for a person to enter into the path of meditation, he or she must change the way they interact with the world. To accomplish this, an individual needs to focus their attentions in a new and more refined manner. This oftentimes causes turmoil, however, for the thinking mind of the average individual has been allowed to think what it has wanted to think and the body allowed to consume and partake of what it has craved. Thus, to many individuals, simply beginning to meditate is *Tapasia*.

There have been holy men who, for thousands of years, have put their bodies and minds to the ultimate test in the name of *Tapasia*. There are many who forgo the wearing of clothing, or give up talking. Others, vow to stand on one leg for the rest of their lives. Many retreat to caves, never to interact with other humans again. All of these are extreme examples of *Tapasia*. To the modern practitioner, seeking simply to calm and refine their mind through meditation, this level of excessive *Tapasia* is not required.

*Tapasia* to the modern practitioner is based more upon dismissing the emotional and material excesses that your life has commonly come to embrace. For many, to stop drinking soft drinks or coffee is an intense austerity. To others, simply sitting in meditation two times a day is excessive *Tapas*. Therefore, *Tapas* must be defined by the individual and not measured by what others have previously chosen as their individual practice in this required level of mental and physical discipline.

4. ***Svadhyaya*** means, *"Spiritual study."*

Many individuals falsely believe that they already know all that there is to know. This is based upon personal ego, psychological insecurity, or the desire for a person to believe that he or she is more than they truly are.

Over the centuries many people have walked the spiritual path. From them, we can gain great knowledge and wisdom. Each of the obstacles we individually run up against have been encountered by others who have eventually overcome them, from their paths we can learn how to more quickly bypass these obstacles and realign and rebalance our lives. To this end, *Svadhyaya* is an essential element to each of our ongoing evolution.

5. ***Ishvara Pranidhana*** means, *"God Consciousness"* or *"Supreme Consciousness." Pranidhan* means, *"Surrender to."* Thus, *Ishvara Pranidhana* means, *"Surrendering to God."*

Many modern individuals choose to not believe in the existence of God or a supreme consciousness. They consider this system of belief superstition – believing that all that happens in this world is simply random chaos, set in motion by some not yet defined scientific causation. It is certainly not the objective of this book to attempt to alter anyone's beliefs. Thus, if that is what you believe – that is what you believe. From ancient cultures forward, however, there has existed the belief in a supreme entity. This being or energy has been called untold names and has been assigned a multitude of images. If you believe in a supreme being, by whatever name or form, this is what you surrender your ego, desires, and thinking mind onto. This is the essence of Patanjali's focus for this stage of meditative preparation.

### Perfect Interaction

If we step outside of ourselves for a moment and stop believing that we are the center of the universe, we witness that there is an extremely vast plethora of energies, life forms, and so many perfectly timed cosmic interactions going on, that there must be some source of supreme knowledge which has orchestrated this divine melodrama. Certainly, we as individuals may not like everything that is taking place on this physical plane. But, if we move beyond our own limited perceptions for a second we see that the constant movement of the waves, the flowing of the rivers to the sea, the ever changing seasons, the construction and destruction of surface by the elements of nature is overwhelmingly amazing and it all happens with such a perfection that there must be a cosmic maestro.

You are an individual participant of this divine perfection. You have a purpose to serve or you would not be here. If you choose to be unhappy, you can be unhappy. If you choose to pursue enlightenment, you can. It is all your choice, defined only by the placement you have received in this cosmic theater. Surrender to it and you are free. You do what you do, seeing all action as your pathway to closer connection to God or *Cosmic Consciousness*. From this belief, you no longer resist and make yourself uncomfortable and miserable. Instead, you become a conscious player in this grandiose theater of life.

## Chapter 5
## Asana
*The Seat of Meditation*

Asana is the third level of Pantajali's *Astanga Yoga. Asana,* translated from the Sanskrit, means *"Seat or Throne."* In the modern era this word is commonly used to describe the physical postures practiced in *Hatha Yoga.* In classic yoga, however, this word describes a firm meditative posture whereby the individual who meditates could sit for long periods of time and meditate undisturbed by the external world.

The classic posture for seated meditation is *Padma Asana* or the *Lotus Pose.* This is where the practitioner sits cross-legged on the ground.

There are three variations of this posture. The first and most basic is *Sukh Asana.* This is where the legs are naturally crossed and the feet touch the ground underneath the thighs. The second, *Arddha Padma Asana "Half Lotus,"* is where the top of one foot is brought up and placed on the thigh of the opposite leg. The third, *Padma Asana "Full Lotus,"* is where the right foot is placed on the left thigh and the left foot is placed upon the right thigh.

For centuries it has been taught that *Padma Asana* is the most beneficial posture to assume while meditating. It is stated in ancient texts that this pose naturally stimulates the spinal nerves that activates the energies of the body.

Though this is the traditional posture for meditation, it is unduly uncomfortable for many individuals. If this discomfort is based upon your lack of desire to sit on the floor in this position, then you should make the practice of this posture one of your *Tapasia* and master the pose. If, on the other hand, you cannot sit in this pose comfortably due to arthritis in your hips or knees, then you should sit in whatever position you can comfortably maintain for an extended period of time, with your spine straight, as you practice meditation.

# Chapter 6

*Pranayama*
*Breath Control*

The forth stage of Patanjali's *Eightfold Path of Astanga Yoga* is *Pranayana*. Modern science teaches us that every element of this universe, from the smallest subatomic particle to the largest planet is vibrating with energy. In Sanskrit, that energy is known as *"Prana,"* which means *"Vital Force."*

Your human body continually pulsates with *prana*. Those individuals who have large amount of *prana* are energetic, happy, and vital. Those with low amounts of *prana* are lethargic, sad, and depressed.

*Prana* is regulated in your body by your breath. Therefore, excess amounts of *prana* can be brought into your body through precise breath control techniques. These techniques are known as, *"Pranayama."* Through the practice of *pranayama* your physical and emotional being is enhanced as well as your mind can be guided into meditative states.

### Energy Movement

It is understood that *Prana* emanates through the human invisible via invisible energy channels. In Sanskrit these channels are known as, *"Nadis."* For a person to remain healthy it is understood that *prana* must be allowed to travel uninhibited via these channels. This understanding is the same concept used by acupuncturists who refer to *prana* as *"Chi"* or *"Ki."*

### Nadis

There are seventy-two thousands *nadis* acknowledged in the human body. Of these, three are the most important to the meditative practitioner. These three channels are: *Sushmuna, Pingala,* and *Ida.*

### Sushmuna Nadi

*Sushmuna Nadi* is the, *"Most Gracious Channel."* It is located central to the spine – traveling from the base to the top of the head. As it is the primary canal where *pranic* energy flows, it is considered the most important of all the *nadis* of the human body. This *nadis* is the primary pathway where *prana* travels upwards in the human body. This channel is sometimes referred to as *"Moksha Marga"* or *"The way to liberation."*

### Pingala Nadi

*Pingala Nadi* or the *"Sunrise Current"* travels to the right of *Sushmuna Nadi*. It rises from the base of the spine and exits at the right nostril. This current is responsible for heating the body. A practical experiment that can be performed to demonstrate the effectiveness of *nadis* understanding is, the next time you are cold while sleeping, lay on your left side. This will cause your body to naturally begin breathing predominately through your right nostril. Thus, activating the *Sushmuna Nadi*. You soon will begin to feel much warmer.

## Ida Nadi

*Ida Nadi* or the *"Channel of Comfort"* is located to the left of the *Sushmuna Nadi*. This pathway rises from the base of the spine and ends at the left nostril.

*Ida Nadi* is the cooling current of the body. As was the case with the previous *Sushmuna Nadi* experiment, you can simply lay on your right side if you are feeling too warm and activate *Ida Nadi*. You will immediately begin to cool down.

## Pranayama and Meditation

There are literally hundreds of *pranayama* techniques that have been developed over the centuries that are used to activate very specific elements in the human form. There are three primary *pranayama* techniques used in association with yoga meditation, however. Both of these techniques are used to calm the mind of the practitioner in order to more easily reach a state of meditation, they are: *Deergha Swasam, Sukha Purvaka,* and *Nadi Sudi.*

## Deergha Swasam

The most basic level of *pranayama* teaches you to simply take in a few very deep breaths and guide these breaths deeply into your abdomen. This technique is known in Sanskrit as, *"Deergha Swasam."* Literally, *"Deep Breathing."* This simple *pranayamic* exercise will greatly revitalize you your mind and cause you gain instant mental focus. This simple exercise will additionally provide you with an immediate dose of *prana*. From this, you can move forward with your practice of meditation in a much more focused and invigorated manner.

In fact, you should practice this exercise, of taking a few deep breaths, several times every day simply to cleanse your lungs of impurities and realign your inner being with the cosmic energy of *prana*.

### Sukha Purvaka

The *pranayamic* breath that will actually aid you in your meditation is *Sukha Purvaka*. *Sukha Purvaka* means, "The Easy Breath," in Sanskrit.

*Sukha Purvaka* is designed to quickly calm your mind and lower your cardiovascular rate in order to prepare you to enter into a meditative mindset. This breath is known to invoke a clear and positive state of mind.

To begin this exercise, sit down in a comfortable position. Close your eyes, straighten your spine. Watch your breath naturally come in and then leave your body. Mentally, embrace the life giving force of each breath.

When you feel that you are ready, close off your right nostril with your right thumb. Breathe slowly and naturally in through your left nostril. When your in-breath is complete, naturally allow this breath to leave your body, also through your left nostril.

Perform this exercise for twelve breaths. When you have completed your final exhalation, place your right hand back down in your lap, raise your left hand, and close off your left nostril for the same twelve natural breaths. When you have completed this repetition, place both hands in your lap and mentally focus for a few moments before your begin your meditation session.

From this exercise, not only will you rise in a very calm state of mind but your mental clarity will be extremely focused, as well.

### Nadi Sudi

*Nadi Sudi* means, *"The Nerve Purifying Breath."* This breathing exercise is an essential body and mind calming technique. There is no *pranayamic* technique more well suited to quickly calming your racing mind and slowing your accelerate heart rate. *Nadi Sudi* quickly brings about a lightness of body and a calm and focused mind. It is an ideal technique to perform just prior to entering into meditation.

To begin *Nadi Sudi,* sit down. As you cannot immediately rush into a meditative state of mind, allow yourself to relax and reflect for a few moments. When you feel you are ready, close your eyes and take a deep breath. Hold this in-breath for as long as is comfortable and then consciously release it.

Place your right hand up to your nose. By pushing against the right nostril with your thumb, close it off. Breathe slowly, yet deeply, in through the left side of your nose. Observe your breath enter and slowly flowing into your body in a stream of calming energy. Once your in-breath is complete, allow it to remain in your lungs for five seconds. Slowly count, *"One, two, three, four, five."* Now, open your right nostril by removing your thumb from it. At the same time, close your left nostril by placing your forefinger against it. Allow the breath to, slowly and naturally, flow out from your body through your right nostril. Once your breath has completely exited, feel the serene emptiness. Count, *"One, two, three, four, and five."*

When it is time to breathe in, take the breath in through your right nostril. Hold it, as previously described, for the count of five. When the time of breath release has come, close off your right nostril with your thumb, opening your left nostril, and allow the breath to slowly exit via your left nostril.

Repeat this process approximately twenty times. This exercise is a calming breathing technique that allows you not only quiet your racing thoughts but also additionally refocuses your mind on the process of meditation.

# Chapter 7
## Pratyahara

*Pratyahara* is the fifth level of *Astanga Yoga*. It details that the meditative practitioner should withdraw his senses from the external world and embrace *"Non-being."*

Non-being is an abstract consciousness. In the modern world we have all been programmed to identify ourselves with the thought of *"I." "I am a human being." "I look like this." "I feel this way at this particular moment." "I think this about that." "I want that, right now."* and so on. Though this is what we have been trained to accept as normal consciousness, the individual on the path of consciousness attempts to step past this limited perception of life.

**Desire and Non-being**

How many times have you gone outside and desired an object so much that you completely lost your peace due to the fact that you began to obsess about how you could come to acquire it? How many times have you been outside and you saw a beautiful person that you physically or emotionally wished that you could come to know? How many times have you been watching television or reading a magazine and realized that you truly wished to live the life of a specific person? Why did this desire arise? Because you saw them. If you had not, you would not even know that they existed and you would be one step closer to ultimate peace.

The physical world is infamous for dragging you into desire. This has been the case since the dawn of humanity. *Pratyahara* instructs that you must move away from the distracting influences of the physical world to truly be able to embrace divine consciousness.

*Pratyahara* teaches that you must remove yourself from the false precipice motivated by external visual and sensory stimuli in order that you may embrace the non-being nature of divine consciousness. To achieve this, you must retreat from the world.

To some, this has meant escaping to live in caves or monasteries. *Pratyahara* does not have to be that extreme, however.

To practice *Pratyahara,* within the constraints of modern society, you can do something as simple as setting aside a certain portion of home where you consciously will not allow desires or desire stimulating objects to enter. This location does not have to be grandiose. It can be a designated corner of your home. A location where you can every day you will go to this quiet location and consciously withdraw your senses from desire.

The path of *Pratyahara* is not instantaneous. As is the case with all forms of meditation, it must be practiced. As such, it is important to keep in mind that when you go to this location you will not instantly fall deeply into desireless meditation simply because you have entered the space and have sat down. Entering this area, however, will certainly be a motivating precursor to the falling away of desire and meditation.

**Pratyahara Practice**

Once you have seated yourself in this location, you will quiet your mind by consciously removing your thoughts from the luring aspects of the material world. Mentally see all the desires you possess fall away. Witness the sensation of your body and mind not desiring anything. Without desire, witness your mind merge into the oneness of the cosmic whole. See yourself as a non-entity, pure energy.

# Chapter 8
## Dharana

*Dharana* is the sixth stage of Patanjali's *Eightfold Path of Astanga Yoga*. The Sanskrit word *Dharana* means *"Collectedness."* This word is used to define the segment of yoga that involves consciously training your mind to turn off the never-ending racing of thoughts and focusing upon a singular subject. *Dharana* is synonymous with concentration.

### Concentration

Concentration is the predecessor to meditation. It is the necessary forerunner because of the fact that the primary hindrance to meditation is that the mind of the average individual is quickly swayed from any internal focus by the stimuli of the physical world; namely: fantasies, desires, emotions, lust, and so on. Without the ability to clearly focus, meditation is impossible. Thus, the mind must be trained to become *Ekagrata "One-pointed."*

### Sensory Overload

The problem exists, in the modern world that the majority of its population is living on sensory overload. There are continued tasks to accomplish, bills to pay, relationships to cultivate, and desires to be fulfilled. Without formal training, it is virtually impossible to pull your mind away from the thoughts that go hand-in-hand with all of these worldly pursuits and sit down and meditate.

Many people who attempt to go straight into meditation, with out the necessary prerequisite of *Dharana,* are immediately disheartened due to the fact that their mind is constantly wandering and they believe that they are incapable of truly meditating. This is not the case. Your mind simply needs to be trained to acutely focus and concentrate. Once it is learned that you can truly focus, meditation will come naturally and there will not be the demeaning inner dialogue rebuking yourself for not being able to sit for more than a few seconds without having a million thoughts overpowering your concentration.

### Creating Concentration

To simply sit down and turn off your thoughts is virtually impossible. From birth forward we have continually been indoctrinated into the process of thinking. In fact, not thinking seems quite unnatural.

As you begin on the path of yoga meditation you must initially learn how to harness your thoughts. You cannot harness your thoughts by simply sitting down and mentally telling yourself to, *"Stop thinking."* You may be able to hold your focus for a moment or two but then the memory of a past occurrence will pop into your mind or the idea of a desired person or possession comes into your thoughts. Before you know it, your mind has entered into the realm of pure fantasy and your meditative hopes are lost. To remedy this, you must learn how to control your thinking mind and train it to precisely focus.

From the ancient techniques of *Dharana* you will begin to quickly see results and you will no longer be dominated by racing thoughts. Thus, you will gradually be able to enter into a true meditative mindset.

## The Techniques of Dhrana

There are several highly effective techniques that have been developed over the centuries that will help you calm your racing mind. You can work with a single technique or multiple techniques until you find the one that is most beneficial to you.

## Tratak

*Tratak* is the *Dharana* exercise of *"Focused Gazing."* It is stated in the ancient Hindu scripture known as The Vedas, *"Where the eye goes, so follows the mind."* This is the premise behind this concentration technique.

There are three slightly varying methods of *Tratak*. The first is, *"Candle Gazing."*

## Candle Gazing

To perform this *Tratak* you light a candle in a darkened room, sit a few feet in front of it, in a meditative cross-legged posture, and begin to stare. Instead of letting your mind drift off to thoughts, focus your attention upon the candle.

As you will immediately notice, the flame of the candle is in continual motion. The colors change and so does the pattern of the flame. This subtle movement allows you to hold your focus. As it is not a stagnate object, your mind will be drawn into the play of movement the flame unleashes. Each time a thought comes to your mind while you are performing *Tratak,* simply mentally redirect your focus towards the flame – refocus your attention and let go of the thought.

As you perform the *Candle Gazing Exercise* your eyes are not required to remain open. As your concentration abilities intensify, you can periodically decided to close your eyes. When you do this, do not release the image of the burning candle from your mind. Instead, view it in your mind's eye, witnessing the changes that take place in the flame as if your eyes were still open. When the image begins to fade from your mental picture, reopen your eyes and again formalize your physical focus.

When you begin the practice of *Tratak,* you should perform *Candle Gazing* for approximately ten to fifteen minutes. As your mental focus increases, you can extend this time period up to half an hour or longer as you deem appropriate.

## Yantra

*Yantra* is a Sanskrit word that means *"Device."* A *Yantra* is a meditative focal pattern containing geometric images symbolizing human life interacting with *Cosmic Consciousness.* These illustrations provide the meditative practitioner with a focus of concentration.

There have been numerous *Yantra* created over the centuries. Some of them are simple lined representations while others are elaborate interconnected artistic drawings. In either case, as a meditative practitioner you perform the same style of starring exercise as described in the *Candle Gazing Exercise.*

Examples of *Yantras* can readily be found on the Internet or in a spiritual center or bookstore.

To perform *Yantra* concentration, place your visual attention upon the *Yantra,* refusing to think about anything else. Due to the intermingling geometric images, your mind will be drawn into the play of the artistic movement. As your mental focus becomes clearer, you can close your eyes and internalize the image. From this, not only is your concentration deepened but also you will gain insight into the complex interactive movement of human life in association with the cosmic movement of art creations

## Mandala

*Mandala* is a Sanskrit term that means *"Orb"* or *"Sphere."* A *Mandala* is a religious artwork. Though similar to a *Yantra,* a *Mandala* is much more elaborate in composition and structure.

Again, examples of *Mandalas* are readily found on the Internet or at spiritual centers or bookstores.

*Mandalas* can be very beautiful works of art. They are composed of concentric circles that are designed to represent the various levels of human and spiritual consciousness. At the center of a *Mandala* is the *Bindu.* The *Bindu* is the central point of the *Mandala.* From a metaphysical perspective, the B*indu* represents *"The Point"* where human consciousness and absolute reality become one.

As a method of *Tratak, Mandalas* are used in the same fashion detailed in the previous two gazing exercises. You focus your concentration upon the image until it becomes internalized. If your mind begins to wander, you simply refocus your concentration on the artistic image and bring your mind back to a state of thoughtlessness.

As you advance with your use of a *Mandala,* as was the case with the previous two exercises, begin to close your eyes as the spiritual essence of the *Mandala* takes over your thinking mind.

The ideal practice time for both *Yanta* and *Mandala* gazing is to begin with fifteen-minute intervals. As you concentration abilities progress, you can increase the time to up to half an hour.

### Counting: One, Two

For those of you who are limited by environmental constraints or are not internally drawn to the previously detailed *Tratak* exercises, there is a very basic, yet exceedingly effective method for developing acute concentration. This exercise requires nothing more than your sitting down in a relatively quiet environment, closing your eyes, taking in a few deep breaths to cleanse your lungs of any impurities and substantiate your connection to *pranic energy,* and then guiding your mind to begin watching the incoming and the outgoing of your breathing.

A breath comes in, you count, *"One."* A breath goes out, you count, *"Two."* A new breath come in, you count, *"One."* The breath goes out, you count, *"Two."*

This method of *Dharana* has been adopted by the Zen Buddhists and is referred to in Buddhism as *Zazen. Zazen* means, *"To sit in Zen."*

As you perform this *Dharana* exercise do not attempt to force your breathing in any way. Simply allow the breath to naturally enter and exit your body. At any point you find your mind wandering off to thoughts, refocus your concentration on your breathing and count, *"One," "Two."*

This *Dharana* exercise should be practiced for approximately fifteen minutes a day, at the outset. As you will not want to keep looking at a clock to time yourself, it is a good idea to set a soft alarm that will inform you when your session is over. As time progresses, your focus will become much more precise. With this, you can extend the period of your *"Sitting"* for as long as you feel is appropriate.

## Mastering Dharana

The techniques of *Dharana* are specifically designed to focus your mind. When you first begin their practice, you will, no doubt, periodically wander off to the random thinking process that has been present throughout your life. This is not unnatural and you should not rebuke yourself because of it. Simply, catch yourself, refocus your attention on your chosen *Dharana* technique and continue its practice. After you have performed *Dharana* for a few months, you will one day conclude a session and will be amazed to find that your mind was not driven to indiscriminate thinking at all. As time and your *Sadhana* progresses, you will truly become the controller of your thoughts.

## Chapter 9
# Dhyana

*Dhyana* is the Sanskrit word for meditation. This is the seventh stage of Patanjali's *Eightfold Path of Astanga Yoga.*

### Understanding Meditation

Once you have developed the ability to clearly focus your mental concentration, through the techniques of *Dharana,* you will then possess the ability to take the next step and begin to truly meditate.

The difference between *Dharana* and *Dhyana* is that in meditation your one-pointed mental focus now possesses the ability to be precisely placed upon the deeper realms of reality. From this, you can consciously transcend the limitations and illusions of this physical world and begins to interact with your true inner-self and the cosmic energy that is the essence of this universe.

### Sitting for Meditation

As explained, the cross-legged *Padma Asana* posture has been detailed, throughout the centuries, as the best pose to sit in for meditation. This is because it is known to *"Lock"* the body. From this, *pranic energy* is not allowed to escape.

Additionally, as *prana* rises up the *Nadis* *"Channels"* parallel to the spine during meditation, it is very important that your spine remain erect as you meditate. *Padma Asana* causes your spine to naturally remain upright.

Though this is the ideal posture for meditation, sitting in this position is very uncomfortable for some people. If this is your case, it is fine to meditate in another, more appropriate, positioning for your body type. For example, you can sit in a firm, straight-backed, chair. This will cause your spine to remain erect and, thus, the rise and fall of *prana* will not be hampered.

The most important thing to remember when choosing an alternate meditating posture is to never sit in a location where your spine will have the ability to slouch over or you will be prone to become too comfortable and fall asleep. Easy chairs and couches are never the ideal location to meditate.

## Ama Drishti

When you begin to meditate, closing your eyes is the best method. In Sanskrit this is called *Ama Drishti, "Moon Gazing."*

With your eyes shut, you will not be distracted by any visual stimuli. As meditation, especially at the early stages, can still be confounded by your racing mind, it is important not to add disruptive elements to the process. Thus, meditating with your eyes closed is an essential preliminary technique.

# Chapter 10
## Mudra

The Sanskrit word M*udra* means, *"To seal."* When used in association with meditation, *Mudra* teaches you to hold your hands in a specific position in order to cause *prana* to circulate through your body in a very specific pattern and to bring about a specific type of meditative energy.

There are over thirty *Mudras* used by various Yoga sects, each believed to bring about a clearer meditative focus. Of these, there are four that are most common: *Jnana Mudra, Dhyana Mudra, Anjali Mudra, Abhaya Mudra* and *Shan Mukhi Mudra*.

### Jnana Mudra

*Jnana Mudra* or the *"Seal of Wisdom"* is perhaps the most commonly used *Mudra* in association with meditation. This *Mudra* has you bring the tip of your thumb into contact with the tip of your first finger, forming a circle. Your other fingers are left naturally extended. The top of your hands are then placed upon your knees. This *Mudra* is known to keep *pranic energy* in a pattern of continual circulation within your body.

The reason this *Mudra* denotes wisdom is that the thumb represents the higher self, known in Sanskrit as *"Brahman."* The first finger represents the individual self or *"Atman."* When the two are joined they form a pattern of transcendence where the individual self merges with the universal self, leading to enlightenment.

### Dhyana Mudra

*Dhyana Mudra* is the *"Seal of Meditation."* Laying your left, open palm, in your lap and then placing your right, open palm, loosely on top of it, perform this *Mudra*. The tips of the two thumbs are allowed to touch one another.

This is an easy and very natural *Mudra* to perform and can be used in association with either *Dharana* or *Dhyana*.

### Anjali Mudra

*Anjali Mudra* or the *"Prayer Hands"* is also known as *Namaskara Mudra*. This is a common *Mudra* not only for meditation but it is additionally used when one greets another person of spiritual personage. The *Anjali Mudra* witnesses you put your hands together in prayer position and place them at chest level directly in front of your heart. This *Mudra* is used to invoke a devotional state of mind.

### Abhaya Mudra

*Abhaya Mudra* or the *"Seal of Fearlessness"* is the *Mudra* that dispels fear -- both in the physical and spiritual sense. This *Mudra* is performed by resting your open left hand across your lap. Your right hand is then raised, with your open palm facing outwards. Your fingers are extended upwards in a natural pattern.

This *Mudra* is a posture of strength. It is utilized when a Yogi feels that there is eminent physical or ethereal danger and he wishes to ward off any possible peril.

### Shan Mukhi Mudra

*Shan Mukhi Mudra,* literally means, *"Six Opening Seal."* This is the most elaborate of all *Mudras.* It witnesses you close your eyes, then place your fully open hand upon your face. Your thumbs go in your ears, your first fingers hold your eyes shut, your second fingers close off your nose, and your third and forth finger keep your mouth from opening. Once your hand has been situated upon your face and just prior to closing off your nostrils, take in a deep breath and then close them off. Hold this breath for as long as is comfortably possible. When you find you must exhale, release the breath by lifting your finger off of your nose just slightly. Breathe in, and again close off your nose. This process goes on for as long as you wish to utilize this *Mudra.*

This *Mudra* is known as a technique of *Pratyahara, "Sensory Withdrawal."* It quickly reveals to the meditative practitioner how they are dominated by external stimuli and how they must retreat from these influences if they hope to truly enter into a state of meditation.

## Chapter 11
## Meditative Focus

The *Anja Chakra* or *Third Eye* is the most powerful meditation focal point. Focusing on this *Chakra* is known in Sanskrit as *Tri Shankhi Vajri*.

The power of this location can easily be witnessed. If you calm your mind, close your eyes, and begin to meditate, you will find that your internal gaze is naturally drawn to this energy center. This occurs because of the fact that *Anja Chakra* is the communication point between the human being and the forces that exist in the Astral Realm. Additionally, *Ajna Chakra* is the source point for the *Pranava Mantra*. The most profound *Mantra*, "Om."

It is suggested that this is the point you place all of your meditative focus upon if you hope to achieve *Self-Realization*. Though other *Chakras* may be used to activate specific bodily or astral energies, this is the focal point that guides an individual towards *Cosmic Consciousness*.

## Chapter 12

## Mantra

The Sanskrit root of the word *Mantra*, is *"Man,"* which means *"To think."* The suffix, *"Tra"* means, *"To implement."* Combined, *Mantra* means to implement a very specific type of thought that invokes the essence of divine cosmic energy.

As a meditative practice a *Mantra* is a sacred sound, word, or passage recited by the meditative practitioner, either mentally or verbally, in order to create a meditative state of mind. From this they can come into contact with the cosmic essence of the universe.

### Sanskrit

A *Mantra* is composed of a word or words based in the Sanskrit language. Sanskrit is an ancient dialect believed to be of sacred origins. The root of the word Sanskrit is, *"Samshrta,"* meaning refined, polished, and made perfect.

From a Linguistic standpoint, the origins of Sanskrit can be traced to approximately 1200 B.C.E. Sanskrit is a highly inflected language, with elaborate noun, adjective, and verb morphologies. The words that make up this language are believed to express the true essence or pure meaning of a word. For this reason, traditionally the meditative practitioner or yoga only practices *Mantras* based in the Sanskrit language.

### Mantra Meditation

The reciting of a *Mantra* is one of the most elementally important forms of meditation. Not only does it serve as an advanced method of focusing the mind, but also the essence of the *Mantra* one recites comes to define the inner nature of their being. If the *Mantra* you recite is based on peace, peace is what you emanate. If your *Mantra* is focused upon internal strength, power is what you project. If the essence of your *Mantra* is universal wisdom, understanding becomes the source of your being.

### Japa

*Japa* means repetition. *Japa* is the meditative practice of continually repeating a specific *Mantra*.

To aid in the practice of *Japa,* the meditative practitioner often times uses a *Mala*. A *Mala* is a stand of 108 prayer beads that the practitioner uses as a method to focus his or her meditative concentration upon.

To use a *Mala,* each time you recite your *Mantra* you pass a bead between your thumb and the first finger of your right hand. When the final bead or *Meru* is reached, the *Mala* is turned around and you continue your meditation – passing a bead through your fingers with the pronunciation of each *Mantra*.

Due to its repetitive nature, as you perform *Japa* you may find yourself in a deeper level of internal thinking than you have previously experienced. Though the *Mantra* is automatically repeating in your mind, you may catch yourself thinking about some issue or mentally visualizing some fantasy. This is not unnatural. If this occurs, simply catch yourself, refocus your attention upon your *Mantra,* and bring your concentration back to this pathway to refined consciousness.

### Pranava

*Pranava* is the most sacred *Mantra.* It is the pure eternal sound that radiates throughout this universe. To the human, it is pronounced as, *"Om."*

The prefix of *Pranava* is symbolic of *Prakriti.* This Sanskrit words means, *"Nature."* The suffix is *Nava,* which means, *"Ship."* Together, *Pranava* means, *"The ship which crosses the ocean of human existences and merges the meditative practitioner with the essence of nature and God."*

The *Mantra, "Om"* is sometimes written in English as *"AUM."* This is because of the fact that in Sanskrit, *Om* represents *Trimurti,* the three fundamental components of universal existence, expressed by the Hindu deities: *Brahma,* the creator, *Vishnu,* the preserver, and *Shiva* the destroyer.

Symbolic, *Trimurti* portrays that in life our physical bodies are created – we live, then we die. *Om* embraces this universal truth in a singular statement. As the English written translation, *Om,* does not clearly represent these three states, the spelling is periodically changed.

### Ah

The *Mantra, "Ah,"* is the seed sound that represents the unborn nature of the universe. Ah, is the source of all sound and creation. Ah is what you hear when you listen to the ocean waves, the source of all human life, crashing upon the shore.

### Tat Twam Asai

*Tat Twam Asai,* literally translated from the Sanskrit means, *"I am that."* This refers to the fact that we all possess the divine spirit within us and that we all have the ability, through purification, to become a clear reflection of cosmic understanding.

While reciting this *Mantra* the practitioner reaffirms, *"I am that."* This statement is not made from a state of arrogance. Instead, it is recited as a method to link the subconscious mind with the divine essence present in all of us. With this, the ego-based mind of the practitioner eventually falls away and *Divine Consciousness* is encountered.

### Sat Nam

*Sat Nam,* literally translates as, *"Truth Name."*

Absolute Truth, *"Sat,"* is one of the primary elements of yoga. It must be embrace in order to encounter *Cosmic Consciousness.* Truth, in this sense, is not simply limited to, *"Not lying"* when you speak with others. Though this, of course, is an important basis to begin your understanding of universal truth. To the meditative practitioner, *"Sat"* is known to be one of the primary components that forms the embodiment of the cosmic essence of this universe. Therefore, by repeating the *Mantra, "Sat Nam,"* the zealot transcends the thinking mind where psychological constraints cause the individual to be removed from the truth that we all know as enlightenment and can ascend to a plane of pure consciousness where absolute truth and *Self-Realization* manifests.

### Om Shanti

The Sanskrit word, *Shanti* means *"Peace."* Inner peace is one of the primary elements of *Self-Realization*. Without inner peace the mind rushes from one fixation to the next, emotions dominate the spirit, and the individual is left bound by the chaotic world of desires.

The reciting of, *"Om Shanti,"* not only calms your mind but links you to the pure essence of peace. Thus, it is a very important *Mantra* to use not only in times of stress but as a means to actualize your true essence, which is peace.

### Hamsa Mantra

The deity *Hamsa* is an incarnation of the Hindu God *Vishnu. Hamsa* also can be defined as, *"Swan,"* the symbol of spiritual achievement. The *Mantra, "So Ham," (pronounced Hum)* means, *"I am he."* This *Mantra* is used to invoke the quality of spiritual attainment.

### Ram Nam

*Ram Nam* or *"Name of Ram,"* is a *Mantra* that causes your inner being to project strength and self-confidence.

*Ram* or *Ramachandra* is an incarnation of the Hindu God *Vishnu.* The Hindu scriptures entitled, *The Ramayana* was written about this great warrior and his exploits.

As he is an incarnation of God and a powerful warrior, by reciting his name not only are you performing an act of devotion but also you are activating an unstoppable force within yourself that will guide you towards your goal of *Self-Realization*.

### Sita

*Sita* is the wife of *Rama*. As a goddess she is worshipped as all that is right and good in womanhood and motherhood. When her name is recited, the essence of nature or *Prakriti* is invoked. Her name can also be used in association with *Ram's:* "*Ram Ram Sita Ram.*" This *Mantra* brings male and female energy together, forming a positive union.

### Om Namah Shivaya

The *Mantra*, "*Om Namah Shivaya*" invokes the power of the Hindu God *Shiva*. *Shiva* is the destroyer of ignorance, self-deception, and any blockage between the individual and enlightenment.

### Om Namo Saraswati Nami

The Hindu goddess *Saraswati* is the bestower of wealth. This *Mantra* can be used to activate her divine grace and bring not only material but also spiritual riches into your life.

### Choosing a Mantra

It is important to keep in mind when you go about choosing a *Mantra* that you pick one that you feel closely associated with. The factors that will lead you to this conclusion may involve the type of energy you wish to involve in your life or the style of meditation you are most drawn to. It may take some experimentation on your part to find the *Mantra* which you feel most comfortable with. Once you are certain that a specific *Mantra* is the proper one for you, it is very important that you no longer shift your focus trying various *Mantras*. To do this creates a disturbance of energy in your inner and outer being – as each *Mantra* is very specific in the type of consciousness it invokes. As such, the benefits of *Mantra* meditation will not be experienced if your mind is like a yo-yo, juggling various types of energy.

Certain *Mantras* such as *"Om Shanti"* or *"Ram"* can be used to create a certain type of mindset that may be needed in a specific segment of your life. But, when it is time for you to return to formal meditation, then you must refocus on one specific, predetermined, *Mantra*.

### Mantra Initiation

Throughout the centuries it has been taught that it is best to be initiated into a *Mantra* by a *Guru*. This is because of the fact that a *Guru* possesses the wisdom to assign you the proper *Mantra* to aid in your karmic evolution, as you step towards enlightenment. Initiation is not always possible, however. As such, you should not let this stop you from following this method of yoga meditation.

Note: The practice of yoga meditation was founded around the concepts of the Hindu understanding of reality. For this reason, the *Mantras* of yoga meditation are commonly in the Sanskrit and reflect the energies represented by

Hindu deities. In our modern world many people possess firmly held religious and philosophic belief systems. To some, reciting the name of a Hindu based God, Goddess, or understanding may be unsavory. If this is the case, a *Mantra* can be created reflecting the name of *Jesus, Mohammed,* or another religious or form of energy that you deem worthy of meditative focus.

## Chapter 13
## Brahmamurti

Traditionally, in monastic India, a meditative practitioner will rise to meditate in the time period known as *Brahmamurti, "The Hours of God."* This begins each day at 4 A.M. and formal seated meditation continues until 5:30 or 6:00 A.M.

The reason this time period is utilized is that it is believed to be the most, *"Silent,"* time of the day – predawn, before the average person has awakened. It also allows the practitioner to be in a state of refined consciousness when the sun comes over the horizon. Thus, allowing him or her to be fueled by the powerful energy of the life giving sun, known in Sanskrit as *Surya.*

Though this is the ideal time to meditate, for some it is not possible to rise at this early hour in the morning due to jobs, families, and so on. Though you may not be able to meditate during *Brahmamurti,* it is essentially important to set a very specific time when you will meditate every day – as the deepening of meditation is highly enhanced by structure.

Though meditation is available to you at any time, it is imperative that you train your body and mind to enter into this cosmic interactive mindset at a prescribed time period each day.

The amount of time you meditate is not carved in stone. When you begin, you may only sit for ten or fifteen minutes. As your meditation deepens you may find yourself sitting for a half hour, up to one hour, or more.

# Chapter 14
## Samadhi

The eighth and final stage of Patanjali's *Eightfold Path of Yoga* is *Samadhi* or enlightenment. *Samadhi* literally means *"Ecstasy"* in Sanskrit. It is the supreme level of human consciousness. It is understood to be the final step in human consciousness where the individual merges with the divine in a state of all-knowing *Self-Realization* and cosmic awareness.

There are three primary levels of *Samadhi* detailed in the Vedas. The first is *Savikalpa Samadhi*. This is the stage of enlightenment where the individual has focused his attention upon an image of the divine and has merged and become one with this deity or energy. At this level, the person is still aware of his or her human form, yet he or she is not identified with the constrains of personality or worldly desires.

The second level of *Samadhi* is known as *Nirvikalpa Samadhi*. This level of enlightenment witnesses the individual is devoid of self and all levels of bodily consciousness have been replaced by the ecstasy of complete and total divine interaction – *Cosmic Consciousness*.

There is one final type of *Samadhi,* commonly understood to come to the practitioner of meditation on the path to *Self-Realization*. This sage is known as *Sahaja Samadhi*. This is the instantaneous enlightenment that the Zen Buddhists have named *Satori*. This is enlightenment that simply happens. It occurs in an instant of divine insight where the individual self falls away and supreme knowledge is understood. The individual who achieves this is known as a *Jivamukta,* "The living liberated."

**Understanding Enlightenment**

Ultimately, each individual possesses his or her own definition of enlightenment. The primary concept to embrace when coming to terms with a true understanding of enlightenment is that enlightenment is not some far off plateau which is reachable only by the most holy. Instead, enlightenment is your developed ability to encounter each life-event with the understanding that all things that occur to us, while we are in a physical body, happens with a divine purpose. All we have to do is shift our perception of each life-occurrence, step back from our momentary desires for how we want each life event to unfold, and we enter into the space where we understand that life is perfect. All events in life are perfect. Every encounter we have in life is perfect. Giving in to the perfection, enlightenment is no longer an unreachable plateau. Enlightenment become available right here, right now.

From the practice of meditation you are allowed to bring you mind to a clam and focused place, were you are not dominated by desire. This is the source point of encountering the perfection of this world and embracing enlightenment.

# Conclusion

It is important to keep in mind that meditation is not a forced discipline. It is something that you choose to do. If you allow your body, mind, and thoughts to remain in a rebellious and turbulent state, you will never achieve a meditative mindset. But, if you decide to make meditation a part of your life, you consciously take control over your mind and focus your attention.

Begin your practice of meditation with the techniques of *Dharana*. This will guide you into a calmer and more focused state of being. As you move forward, you will find what method of meditation works best for you. From this, you will embrace a sense of mental and physical understanding never encountered by the individual who does not follow the path of meditation. Even if it is only for a few minutes, choose to meditate everyday and the benefits will quickly be self-evident. The practice of yoga meditation will quite you to a new and much more refined sense of tranquility and life-purpose.

## About the Author

Scott Shaw is a prolific author and filmmaker. He is recognized as one of the preeminent Martial Arts Masters of the Western world and is at the forefront of integrating spirituality in the Martial Arts. During his youth he became deeply involved with Eastern Meditative Thought. This guided him to Asia where he has been initiated into Hindu, Sufi, and Buddhist sects. Today, Shaw frequently returns to Asia, documenting obscure aspects of Asian culture in words and on film. He is a frequently featured contributor to Martial and Meditative Art journals and is the author of numerous books on the Martial Arts, Ki Science, Zen Buddhism, Yoga, and Meditation.

## Scott Shaw's *Books-In-Print* include:

*The Little Book of Yoga Breathing,*
*Nirvana in a Nutshell,*
*About Peace: 108 Ways to Be At Peace*
  *When Things Are Out of Control,*
*Zen O'clock: Time To Be,*
*The Tao of Self Defense,*
*Samurai Zen,*
*The Ki Process: Korean Secrets*
  *for Cultivating Dynamic Energy,*
*The Warrior is Silent:*
  *Martial Arts and the Spiritual Path,*
*Hapkido: Korean Art of Self Defense,*
*Taekwondo Basics,*
*Advanced Taekwondo,*
*Chi Kung For Beginners,*
*Essence: The Zen of Everything,*
*Hapkido: Essays on Self-Defense,*
*Zen Buddhism: The Pathway to Nirvana,*
*Zen: Tales from the Journey,*
*Zen in the Blink of an Eye,*
*Yoga: A Spiritual Guidebook,*
*The Little Book of Zen Meditation*

www.ingramcontent.com/pod-product-compliance
Lightning Source LLC
LaVergne TN
LVHW051209080426
835512LV00019B/3183